Healthy by *Design*

Love God, Lose Weight

Freedom from emotional eating,
overeating, and self-sabotage by
accepting God's love

Cathy Morenzie

Guiding Light Publishing

First Edition (as Receiving God's Love): February 2019

Second Edition (as Love, God, Lose Weight): December 2019

ISBN: 978-1-9992207-5-4 (print)
978-1-9992207-4-7 (digital)

Published by Guiding Light Publishing
261 Oakwood Avenue, York, ON, Canada, M63 2V3

Note: The information in this book is for educational purposes only and is not recommended as a means of diagnosing or treating illness. All situations concerning physical or mental health should be supervised by a health professional knowledgeable in treating that particular condition. Neither the author nor anyone affiliated with Healthy by Design dispenses medical advice, nor do they prescribe any remedies or assume any responsibility for anyone who chooses to treat themselves.

Cover Design by: kimmontefortedesign.com

Cover & author photos by http://www.martinbrownphotography.ca/

Interior Design by: Davor Dramikanin

Table of Contents

A Note From the Author

There's a t-shirt that I love to wear that says 'Start with Heart', with a picture of a big heart on the left side of my chest. It reminds me that the starting place of your health journey, or any other life journey for that matter, is with your heart. It means that your heart must be submitted to God if you want to release weight. It means that God is more interested in your heart than what you weigh on the scale, and it means that the condition of your heart will determine your level of success.

And that's why I'm inviting you to (re)start your health journey from a slightly different perspective than you may be accustomed to with other weight loss programs.

Every day, people like you change how they have been approaching their weight loss programs. They share how our *Healthy by Design* books and weightlossgodsway.com online programs have transformed their lives, from reaching their weight goals to increasing their sense of worthiness and self-confidence, while also deepening their relationship with their Heavenly Father.

This book promises to deliver the same results. It will guide and remind you that weight releasing is a heart issue. When you can start with healing your heart by recognizing just how much God loves you, then your success at releasing weight will skyrocket!

And that's what you'll discover when you read this book. You'll discover God's heart for you. You'll discover how you are loved lavishly and passionately by Him. As you read this devotional and challenge, let His love for you fill your every need and desire.

To give you a head start, I'm also offering you these special gifts just for purchasing this book:

Enjoy our Love Letters from God free download. They are designed to help you grasp how wide, how long, how high, and how deep God's love is for you. You can print them out and post them to encourage you and fill you up, use them as a screen saver on your phone or computer, or share them with your friends on social media.

3 Steps to Overcome Emotional Eating – How to overcome emotional eating with God's help. Use this repeatable 3-step approach to reverse impulsive eating habits and turn your needs over to God instead. Join my free newsletter to receive this lesson directly in your inbox and join the 10,000+ Christian women releasing their weight for good, God's Way.

lovegodloseweightbonus.com

Be blessed!

Cathy Morenzie

Cathy

What's Love Got to Do with It?

Tina Turner had a popular song called "What's Love Got to Do with It?".

You may be asking yourself this same question. What *does* love have to do with weight loss?

The answer? Everything!

We do not do the things we want to because we don't feel worthy of having what we want, and it's the love of God that gives us our self-worth.

We don't achieve our goals (weight loss or otherwise) because we're afraid of failing (again), and it's the love of God that affirms us and reminds us that we are enough because we are loved by Him.

We don't stay focused long enough to see results, because we don't have the mindsets and the belief in ourselves to see things through to the end. It's God's love for us that sustains us through the hard times and helps us to fix our eyes on Him and not on our problems. When we look to Him, He only shows us solutions.

When we don't want to do what we know to do, God's love gives us the strength and courage to put one foot in front of the other when we don't feel like moving, when we're paralyzed with fear, and when we don't know what direction we should take.

When we don't understand the process, when we don't know what to do, God's love fills our spirits and saturates us with wisdom and knowledge. He provides us with Godly strategies that we could never have imagined in our own strength.

It's God's love that fills us and encourages us to be the best version of ourselves as He allows us to see ourselves not as we see ourselves or as the world sees us but as He sees us. Whole and complete. Lacking nothing.

The freedom, peace, and joy we're searching for in this life will only come from an understanding and acceptance of God's overwhelming and steadfast love for us.

"Let all that you do be done in love."
(1 Corinthians 16:14 ESV)

- God's love is steadfast and unchanging

- God's love transforms our lives

- God's love comforts us

- God's love is revealed to us through Jesus Christ

- God's love gives us peace and joy

- God's love is poured into us through the Holy Spirit

- God's love compels us to love one another

- God's love heals our broken hearts

- God's love inspires and empowers us

- God's love motivates us

- God's love frees us

In this devotional, you will learn how to give yourself the gift of receiving God's gift of love every day.

Lose Weight, God's Way began as an online Christmas challenge in our weightlossgodsway.com program, and it proved to be so popular we knew we had to make it available to everyone.

This challenge is perfect for any time of year. Spend 10-15 minutes each day receiving God's love from His Word and then doing something kind for yourself.

Remember, you are loved lavishly by God!

What is Healthy by Design?

Healthy by Design (healthybydesignprogram.com) is a series of books, devotionals, challenges, courses and programs all designed to equip women to rely on God as their strength so they can live in freedom, joy and peace.

We understand that there are many factors that keep you from moving from where you are now (overweight, frustrated, overwhelmed, unhappy) to where you want to be (peaceful, free, and joyful) and each devotional will give you the steps to get there.

Each one of our books addresses one aspect of resistance. *Love God, Lose Weight* will help you remove the resistance of low self-esteem.

We call all of these factors 'resistance' because they can potentially strengthen you when you learn how to overcome them. They show up in a variety of forms such as:

- stress
- faulty mindsets
- low self-esteem
- feeling overwhelmed
- poor habits
- lack of faith
- fear of failure

- lack of vision

- other people

- discouragement

However, like going to the gym and performing resistance exercises to strengthen your body, overcoming resistance will make not only your physical body stronger, but also your mind and spirit as well when you discover how to embrace it like James teaches us:

> *"Consider it pure joy, my brothers and sisters, whenever you face trials of many kinds, because you know that the testing of your faith produces perseverance. Let perseverance finish its work so that you may be mature and complete, not lacking anything."*
> (James 1:2–4 NIV)

Healthy by Design will help you to identify what 'resistance' is holding you back, and provide you with the biblical tools as well as practical strategies to help you release the resistance. We show you how to get from where you are now to where you want to be. See the image on the next page.

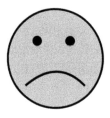

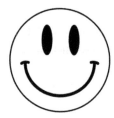

Resistance

stress
faulty mindsets
low self-esteem
overwhelm
poor habits
lack of faith
fear of failure
lack of vision
other people
discouragement

Current

busy
tired
stuck
anxiety
illnesses
stressed
furstrated
no enery
overweight
overwhelmed
dissatisfied with life

Where we want to be

alive
joyful
spirit-led
peaceful
confident
free from illness
healthy weight
boundless energy

Healthy by Design Guiding Principles

1. IDENTIFICATION

Good health is your identity, not your destination.
(Genesis 1:27)

You were created to be in good health. After all, you were created in God's image. Think about that for a minute ... you were created in God's image!

The Bible says, *"Then God said, 'Let Us make man in Our image, according to Our likeness; and let them rule over the fish of the sea and over the birds of the sky and over the cattle and over all the earth, and over every creeping thing that creeps on the earth.' God created man in His own image, in the image of God He created him; male and female He created them."* (Genesis 1:26-27 NASB)

So if that's true, then why have you spent so many years of your adult life trying to get to a specific number on the scale? Just think about the wasted energy, time, frustration, and happiness that you've lost trying to achieve something that you already possess.

The problem is analogous to having an air conditioner on a scorching hot day. We have been given an indispensable tool to help us, but until we plug in the a/c we will never receive the benefit and the power that exists at our disposal. Until we call on the Holy Spirit to be our help, as our instruction book tells us, we will never walk in the authority we have been given.

Soooooo the message here is to:

Stop trying so hard to work at something that you already possess.

Stop being afraid of success. Success is in your DNA—it's who **you are!**

Stop trying to get to a mythical, magical illusion of what you think your life should look like. It's time to see and accept the awesomeness of who you are.

Stop waiting, wishing, wanting, hoping, praying, and wasting time worrying about the future.

I know, easier said than done. But the process starts as you begin to trust that good health is part of your identity, and then stop wasting so much time searching for a magical, mythical reality that does not exist and begin to embrace who God has called you to be—regardless of your current size.

2. TERNION (TRIAD)

*Good health involves a combination of healing
your body, soul, and spirit.*
(1 Thessalonians 5:23)

God made us distinct and unique from all of creation.

Because we were created in God's image, He also created us with a tripartite nature like Himself. As God encompasses the Father, Son, and Holy Spirit, we too are also composed of three parts: our spirit, soul, and body.

As human beings we live in a physical body, we have a soul, and we live eternally as a spirit that connects with God's Spirit. Our tripartite nature works symbiotically together to keep us healthy and whole. It's impossible to address one area without giving attention to the other.

The Bible says, *"Now may the God of peace Himself sanctify you entirely; and may your spirit and soul and body be preserved complete, without blame at the coming of our Lord Jesus Christ."* (1 Thessalonians 5:23 NASB)

For us to be in total health as God intended, all three parts of our being need to be healthy.

They are intertwined and interconnected. Here's how:

Body

Our body is our outer shell, but it houses the temple of the living God. It is your physical being. It consists of our five senses: taste, touch, sight, smell, and hearing. In His infinite wisdom, God created our bodies to operate in harmony with our souls and spirits. If our physical bodies are not healthy, it negatively impacts our spirits and our souls.

Here's what the Bible teaches us about our physical bodies:

It houses the living God (1Cor 3:16-17)

We are to present it to God as a living sacrifice (Romans 12:2)

We are to put no confidence in it (Phil 3:3)

We are to discipline it and keep it under control (1 Cor 9:27)

Soul

Our souls are made up of our conscious and our subconscious mind, which houses our thoughts, conscience, will, and emotions. It gives us our personality. This is where the battle rages. It's where we experience anxiety, doubts, and fears, which in turn manifest in our bodies as excess weight and illness. If our souls are bound then we will have difficulty honoring our temples and we will have difficulty connecting with God.

Here's what the Bible teaches us about our soul:

The Lord created us a living soul. (Gen 2:7)

It is immortal. (Matt 10:28)

It is in conflict with our spirits. (1 Cor 2:14)

They can lead us away and lead to sin and death. (James 1:13-15)

Spirit

At our core is our spirit; it's the part of us that connects with God. This is our contact point with God where our spirit communicates with His. Paul says, "When we cry 'Abba Father', it's the Spirit Himself bearing witness with our spirit that we are children of God." (Romans 8:15-17) It's only when we align our spirits with our Heavenly Father's that we will be ever be successful at anything we do, including getting healthier.

Here's what the Bible teaches us about our spirits:

God enlightens our spirit so we can know truth. (Proverbs 20:27)

The indwelling Spirit of Christ dwells in our heart. (Romans 8:16)

God's Word can divide our souls and spirits. (Heb 4:12)

Key takeaway: We are tripartite beings. Whatever happens to one part of our being has repercussions in the other two areas.

3. REVELATION

Information without revelation is meaningless.
(Romans 8:5 & 12:2; James 1:5)

Here's an obvious, but important question. Do you need more information on weight loss? Didn't think so. You probably already have more information than you can ever read. The problem is not a lack of information but the exact opposite. Most of us suffer from information overload. You probably have books sitting on your bookshelf or table that you mean to read, emails that you need to respond to, or interesting articles that you one day home to skim.

Most women I talk to are so overwhelmed. And I know for sure that the answer they're looking for is not found in reading another book or signing up for another program.

Information in and of itself is meaningless. Ask yourself the following about all the information you've gathered to date:

Revelation comes from the Holy Spirit. It does not come from our wisdom or intellect.. In fact, it's our intellect that keeps getting us into trouble. We 'think' we know more than God, so we keep taking matters back into our own hands. James 1:5 reminds us that it is God who gives us wisdom.

1. Are you applying it?

What good is it to say you trust God with your weight loss yet never submit the journey to Him or never run to Him in your time of need? It's one thing to read something in the Bible or even in a book, but without relying on the power of the Holy Spirit to transform us it's more just information, which has no power on its own. Remember this: 'Knowledge is NOT power; *application* of knowledge is power.'

2. Have you mastered it?

I remember signing up for one of those online 30-day squat challenges. I got up to day four and I quit. Yet if someone asked me, I would probably say, "Yeah, I've done it before." That's what many of us do. We invest in something and quit before we've achieved results, yet we talk like we're now experts on the subject.

I have a similar challenge with tracking my food. Yes I track it, but am I using the tool effectively to eat within my daily allowance or use it as an effective tool for weight management? The answer is 'no', so until then I will continue using it until I learn what I need to learn from the tool. Don't get frustrated or give up if you miss a few days or if you can't stick to it. Keep on trying until you master it.

3. Do your results prove it?

This is the biggest test of true knowledge. I remember striking up a conversation with this marketing 'guru' who began telling me about a new miracle fat-loss pill that has been selling like hot-cakes. He told me all of the benefits of the product and how amazing it was, but he was about 50 pounds overweight! Or have you ever had the sister at church have a Word of the Lord for you, yet her life was in shambles?

Let your results speak louder than your words. Results never lie. If you're not getting results in your weight-loss program, stop wasting time gathering more useless information.

4. TRANSFORMATION

Transformation comes through daily submission.
(2 Corinthians 10:5; Luke 9:23)

Let's face it, sacrificing anything is not pleasant at the time. Even the word itself conjures up feelings of pain and struggle. Yet the Bible teaches us that living a life of sacrifice is the only way to enjoy a life of freedom in Christ. In Matthew 10:39, Jesus says, "Whoever finds his life will lose it, and whoever loses his life for my sake will find it."

The reality is that many of us are frustrated and feel utterly hopeless with our current state of health, but are unwilling to make the necessary sacrifices it takes to achieve a healthy weight. We've been struggling with our weight for most of our lives, and it feels like things will never change. Despite our feelings of hopelessness, we keep grasping at short-term worldly solutions to end our pain. We keep trying solution after solution but they eventually get too difficult, time-consuming, or we just get bored and move on to the next thing.

It's only when we can embrace Jesus' teaching that short-term sacrifice will lead to long-term fulfillment. Then the concept of sacrificial living will not be so daunting.

The solution is found in God. Until we know the true heart of God, sacrifice will always seem like deprivation or punishment. But it's the exact opposite. Freedom is found in dying to ourselves every hour of every day so that we can live an abundant life.

1. God calls us to submission because He understands how easily we are led away by our flesh if we don't exercise restraint.

He knows our propensity to make idols out of everything, and how these idols will turn our attention away from Him.

"No one can serve two masters.
Either you will hate the one and love the other, or
you will be devoted to the one and despise the other.
You cannot serve both God and money."
(Matthew 6:24)

2. God calls us to submission because He knows that our insatiable desires for food (money, power, sex) will always keep us wanting even more. We try to fill our needs with worldly things instead of Godly things, so no matter how much food we eat we will always want more. And no matter how much money we make, we will always want more (Or whatever your weakness is.)

"But each one is tempted when he is carried away
and enticed by his own lust. Then when lust has con-
ceived, it gives birth to sin; and when sin is accom-
plished, it brings forth death..."
(James 1:14-15)

3. God calls us to submission because He knows that He is the only one who can fulfill all of our needs. When we sacrifice our appetites and draw closer to God He honors our actions, meets us in our time of need, and draws closer to us. Satiety and satisfaction are found in Him alone.

"Blessed are those who hunger and thirst for
righteousness, for they will be filled."
(Matthew 5:6)

As you read this book you begin to embrace your weight loss journey as a marathon, not a sprint. You will realize the futility searching for the quick fixes and easy answers, and finally grasp that there is no such thing.

You simply can't cram what the Holy Spirit is trying to teach you on this journey. It's not like a high school test. You're on the journey of your life, and it will take time and patience.

Change is a daily process. It's the little things that you do daily that will get you to your goals.

Every time you say 'yes' to God, you will move closer to your goal.

5. ACTION

"You must move past the natural resistance
from contemplation to action."
(James 1:22 & 2:26)

This principle can be a mouthful so let me take it word by word, starting with the word 'resistance'.

Resistance refers to the trials, roadblocks, difficulties, frustrations, set-backs, and hinderances you encounter on your journey. It could be anything from backsliding, self-sabotage, an injury, an illness in the family, travelling, vacation, family visiting, unexpected company, or anything that slows down or stops your weight loss.

When we experience resistance, most of us usually do one of two things: fight or flight. We either dig our heels in deeper or we quit. What if I told you that none of these options were correct? Resistance is not to be fought. Think of quicksand—the more you resist, the faster you sink. Resistance is to be accepted as part of the natural process. Like going to the gym and performing resistance training exercises to get stronger, you will also discover that resistance can be a good thing.

Next is the word 'contemplation'. Change is part of a process that moves from not being ready to getting ready to being ready to. action. Unfortunately, many of us get stuck and waste years getting ready to get ready but never take action. *Love God, Lose Weight* can help you identify the natural resistance and show you how to jump into action instead of continually procrastinating.

Why participate in this devotional?

For years, Christmas was a time when I'd regrettably gain at least 5-10 pounds. I used the holidays as an excuse to break all my healthy boundaries with the promise that I'd restart my diet on January 1st. This same pattern continued during Valentine's Day, Easter, birthdays, Thanksgiving, and any other celebrations that I felt gave me license to eat.

I only celebrated all the worldly trappings of Christmas and other significant milestones. This often left me feeling empty and in bondage to my uncontrollable habits, so I used even more food to fill the void.

Because I didn't understand that my body was truly God's temple, I manipulated it as I saw fit. I never saw my health as a gift from God or as a responsibility that God had entrusted me to steward, so I did with it as I wanted.

I never realized that losing weight, or any other stronghold in my life, was rooted in emotional issues and, like all emotional issues, could only be healed in the spiritual realm. I did not know that my constant need to stuff myself with food was more about my need to fill my inner emptiness. My overeating was my way to counteract the prevailing feeling of lack.

Over the years I've come to realize that, without a deeper understanding of God's love for me, I'm lost. So, I drew a line in the sand and refused to let Christmas and other events feel like frustrating, overwhelming seasons in my life—over-extended with responsibility and expenses, and over-stuffed with food.

So, one Christmas I decided to start a new tradition during the Advent season, which has made all the difference. And that's why I wrote this devotional.

Each Lenten season (or whenever I need reminders), I study God's word which teaches me just how much God loves me. It has grown and been refined into this 21-day devotional and challenge that will help you to align your heart with the heart of our Heavenly Father's and bring you back to what's most important during your life.

Join me on the journey back to love. That's where our true health, freedom, and peace is found.

As you learn to give and receive God's love, all the other cares of this world will fall away. When love is the foundation of all you do, the Holy Spirit will strip everything else away—even the excess weight!

What will be left is a healthy life of freedom, gratitude, peace, joy, and love rooted in a wonderful relationship with our Heavenly Father.

Although Christmas or Valentine's Day is a great time to participate in this devotional and challenge, God's love is always in season. Which makes this an ideal study for anytime!

If you're tired of constantly gaining and losing weight,

If you want to trust God to help you manage your weight,

If you want to enjoy Christmas or any other holiday without stuffing your body with food and using it as a license to overeat, or

If you want to learn how much God loves you and learn how to ground EVERYTHING you do in this love, then this devotional is for you!

Opening Prayer

Dear Lord, I thank You and praise You that You are love! You don't just 'do' love, You 'are' love! As I begin this three-week devotional and challenge, I give myself over to You entirely. I come to You today with a mind open to transformation and a heart open to receiving the incredible fullness of Your love for me. Help me to set aside a special time each day for us to draw closer. Then safeguard that time from any distraction. I want all I do to be done in love. In the beautiful Name of Jesus, Amen.

Devotions

Day 1

In His Image

Scripture Reflection

"So God created man in His own image,
in the image of God he created him;
male and female he created them."
(Genesis 1:27 ESV)

Can you comprehend what it means to be made in the image of God? Think about it for a minute—it means that you are divinely created. There's no one else like you in all the Earth. Your physical appearance, your personality, your habits, your personal preferences, all these make you one of a kind. Just like no two snowflakes are alike or no two fingerprints are alike, you are uniquely distinguished and set apart from everyone else on this planet.

Too often, we compare our bodies to other people's and wish that we looked like them. Imagine a daffodil wishing it were a tulip. Or a daisy wishing it were a marigold. Sounds ridiculous, right? But that's what we do when we compare ourselves to others. They're all beautiful, they're all unique, and they all bless us because of their differences. God knew what He was doing, and He made you uniquely you. That's something to celebrate!

Today, take a minute and celebrate your uniqueness and divinity.

Today's Love Challenge

Reflect on how God has set you apart and made you unique from anyone else in the world. Share what sets you apart.

_____

_____

_____

_____

_____

_____

_____

_____

Additional Study Scripture

"For those whom he foreknew he also predestined to be conformed to the image of his Son, in order that he might be the firstborn among many brothers."
(Romans 8:29 ESV)

*"And we all, with unveiled face, beholding the glory
of the Lord, are being transformed into the same
image from one degree of glory to another. For this
comes from the Lord who is the Spirit."*
(Romans 8:29 ESV)

1. Reflect on what it means to be created in God's image.
Journal your thoughts.

_____

_____

_____

_____

_____

_____

2. What would your life look like if you truly lived out that
truth?

_____

_____

_____

_____

_____

_____

Today's Prayer

Lord, when I stop to realize that You created the whole world and You saw fit to make me, my mind is blown away! You carefully knitted me together to be uniquely me with a special purpose to fulfill on earth. As I come before You today, I confess that I've cheapened Your workmanship at times by rejecting myself. I am so sorry for this, Lord! I speak the truth that You are good, and that I am fearfully and wonderfully made. I ask Your Spirit to come in and rewire my mind, creating new pathways for me to think about as we go deeper into Your truth over these next weeks. In Jesus' Name, Amen.

Day 2

Transcendent Peace

Scripture Reflection

"Now may the Lord of peace himself give you peace
at all times and in every way."
(2 Thessalonians 3:16 NIV)

One of the most powerful gifts we can manifest is transcendent peace.

This world is anything but peaceful, yet amid all the daily chaos God calls us to be children of peace. How is this possible? Because we serve a living God who loves us with an everlasting love and who offers us peace amid any situation or circumstance. We serve a God who stands in the gap for us and promises to fight for us when necessary.

- No, we're not happy with our weight.

- Yes, we continually eat outside of our boundaries.

- No, we do not have the willpower to stop ourselves from eating the things we don't want to eat.

Despite all these things that threaten to steal our peace, we can still find rest and peace in our Heavenly Father.

God loves us so much, and offers to take our heavy burdens so we can experience His gift of transcendent peace.

As you maneuver through the highs and lows of your days, may you discover the heart of your Heavenly Father to bring you peace each day.

Today's Love Challenge

Find at least 15 minutes today to stop and experience God's peace. Light a candle, read a book, play some music, do something to cultivate a spirit of peace in your life. Write down what you did.

_____

_____

_____

_____

_____

_____

_____

Additional Study Scripture

"You keep him in perfect peace whose mind is stayed
on you, because he trusts in you."
(Isaiah 26:3 ESV)

"For God is not a God of confusion but of peace."
(1 Corinthians 14:33 ESV)

1. The dictionary defines transcendent as 'something so excellent that it's beyond the range of human understanding.' Think about the level of peace that is available to us.

_____

_____

_____

_____

_____

2. What is stealing your peace? Offer it up to God and allow Him to exchange your worries for His gift of peace.

_____

_____

_____

_____

_____

3. Think about the lack of peace that accompanies your health journey—especially during this time of year. Visualize yourself laying it all at His feet. Journal your experience.

_____

_____

_____

_____

_____

_____

_____

_____

Today's Prayer

Dear Jesus, thank You for leaving me the precious gift of Your peace. You have given me an unshifting rock to stand on when the waters get rough, an anchor in every storm, and shelter and protection from every evil. You have left me promises of Your unfailing love. You comfort me, You say that I am the apple of Your eye, You work all things together for my good, and You promise to never leave me. I admit that I can still feel alone at times. I confess today that I cannot bring myself peace and that I desperately need it. So, I'm coming today, praising You for your goodness and love, and asking You for the gift of Your peace to fill my heart. Thank You, Jesus. Amen.

Day 3

His Steadfast Love

Scripture Reflection

> *"Know therefore that the LORD your God is God,*
> *the faithful God who keeps covenant and steadfast*
> *love with those who love him and keep his*
> *commandments."*
> (Deuteronomy 7:9 NIV)

We have all had experiences where someone promised to love us and ended up hurting us. Or someone promised they would do something for us and let us down.

God is not like that. He always keeps his promises. He is always faithful. He will never take His love away from us, no matter how many times we pull away or try to do life without Him. God pursues us with His steadfast, relentless love and wants us to open our hearts to receive it.

Beloved, know that there is nothing you could ever do that can separate you from His love. Despite how many times you break your boundaries, God will never stop loving you. He's not mad at you because you're not walking in the level of health you desire. Yes, He wants you to be healthy because He does not want anything standing in the way of your relationship with Him, but He's not waiting for you to get your act together. He loves you just as you are!

The next time you feel frustrated, alone, lonely, stressed or unloved, remember that you can always turn your heart toward our Heavenly Father and simply receive a fresh anointing of His powerful and steadfast love.

Today's Love Challenge

Think of one thing that you need to forgive yourself for and then forgive yourself.

_____

_____

_____

_____

_____

Additional Study Scripture

"For your steadfast love is before my eyes, and I walk in your faithfulness."
(Psalm 26:3 ESV)

"Your steadfast love, O Lord, extends to the heavens, your faithfulness to the clouds."
(Psalm 36:5 ESV)

1. The dictionary defines steadfast as 'unwavering, loyal, faithful, committed, devoted, dependable, reliable, steady, true, constant.' No person could ever love us like that, but God can. Thank Him.

2. Reflect on God's steadfast love in your life. Think of all the ways He has loved you and journal them.

_____

_____

_____

_____

_____

_____

3. In what ways have you sought love from food, people, or possessions? Repent to God for putting other things before Him, and allow His love to saturate every fiber of your being.

_____

_____

_____

_____

_____

Today's Prayer

Dear Lord Jesus, thank You so much for Your unfailing, steadfast love. I am completely astounded at how You could see me and know everything about me and still love me. You know everything I've ever thought and done, and though it doesn't always honor You, You forgive me and You love me still. Today, I ask for Your help to experience Your love more deeply. Holy Spirit, I invite You now to show me something I'm holding against myself that You've already paid the price for with Jesus' blood. Help me to surrender it totally to You now. Thank You for Your amazing grace and steadfast love. Amen.

Day 4

God's Gift of Patience

Scripture Reflection

*"But you, O Lord, are a God merciful and
gracious, slow to anger and abounding in steadfast
love and faithfulness."*
(Psalm 86:15 ESV)

I'm in constant need of reminders that I am to be patient with myself. I'm constantly getting mad at myself for procrastinating, for not measuring up to an impossible standard that I set for myself, for not having enough willpower, for eating too much, for wasting too much time on the internet when I could be going for a walk, and I could go on and on.

And then I read the Word and I see how patient He is with us. His patience lovingly beckons us back to Him. He gently guides us to simply trust Him and await His direction. What a contrast to my approach.

God's Word teaches me that patience is grounded in love. Because He loves us and has no other agenda, He can be patient with us. Then I see my impatience and I realize it's because I have an agenda. I want results fast, I crave worldly possessions like money and status, or I seek fulfillment in things that don't satisfy me.

Today's Love Challenge

Think of one task that you will accomplish today. Take a moment right now and pray for His Spirit of patience to help you accomplish it. Journal your experience or thoughts after completing this challenge.

_____

_____

_____

_____

_____

_____

Additional Study Scripture

"The Lord is not slow to fulfill his promise as some
count slowness, but is patient toward you,
not wishing that any should perish,
but that all should reach repentance."
(2 Peter 3:9 ESV)

"But you, O Lord, are a God merciful and gracious,
slow to anger and abounding in steadfast love and
faithfulness."
(Psalm 86:15 ESV)

1. Reflect on God's purpose and intention to instill patience in you. How will it bless you?

_____

_____

_____

_____

_____

_____

2. What are you patiently (or impatiently) waiting on from the Lord? Talk to Him about it.

_____

_____

_____

_____

_____

3. Thank God for loving you enough to not give you what you want when you want it, but in His perfect timing.

_____

_____

_____

_____

_____

_____

_____

_____

Today's Prayer

Lord, I pray that I would learn how to cultivate the spirit of patience. Give me Your perspective so that I can focus on what matters most and not waste time striving for results in areas that don't matter anyway. Help me to understand that life is about practice, not perfection, so I may gain a heart of patience and wisdom as You are patient towards me. Teach me how to be patient with myself. I rest in Your peace and patience as You guide me towards Your perfect and pleasing will. In Jesus' Name, Amen.

Day 5

Oh, Give Thanks

Scripture Reflection

> *"Give thanks to the God of heaven, for his steadfast*
> *love endures forever."*
> (Psalm 136:26 ESV)

Thanksgiving is one of the simple ways that we can acknowledge God's provision, power, and providence in our lives. We have much reason to give God thanks because of His steadfast love, His mercy, His kindness, His goodness, and His grace. We serve a living God who is perfectly worthy of all the thanksgiving and praise we can muster up.

When you have a heart of thanksgiving, it's hard to stay down in the dumps or focus on all the things that are not going right in your life. It's hard to hate your body when you are giving God thanks for creating you in His image. Your frustration can quickly turn to gratitude when you give thanks for the food that you're eating and for the ability to move your limbs.

Just one minute of offering praise and thanksgiving to God will create an atmosphere of praise and joy that will quickly change your perspective and your mood.

Today's Love Challenge

Take time to write out a list of all the things that you are thankful for. Give God thanks for everything on your list.

_____

_____

_____

_____

_____

_____

_____

Additional Study Scripture

"I will praise the name of God with a song;
I will magnify him with thanksgiving.
This will please the Lord more than an ox or
a bull with horns and hoofs."
(Psalm 69:30–31 ESV)

"We give thanks to you, O God;
we give thanks, for your name is near.
We recount your wondrous deeds."
(Psalm 75:1 ESV)

1. Reflect on the importance of giving thanks always. Journal your thoughts.

_____

_____

_____

_____

2. Thank God for how He is changing you from the inside out and for guiding you on your weight loss journey.

_____

_____

_____

_____

_____

3. Think about all the things you take for granted. Now give thanks to God for all of them. Does it change your perspective?

_____

_____

_____

_____

Today's Prayer

Dearest Gracious God, I am astounded by Your love! I thank You that You truly are a good, good Father. Lord, I am truly in awe of You for all the ways You have blessed me. Thank You so very much! I want to pour out my praise now, Lord, for all that You are. For Your love and sacrifice. For the breath in my lungs. For the grace and forgiveness that You so freely give. Help me now, Holy Spirit, to focus my mind on all the amazing blessings in my life that have come from You. There is no good apart from You, Lord! In the Name of Jesus, Amen.

Day 6

God's Ultimate Sacrifice

Scripture Reflection

"But God shows his love for us in that while we were still sinners, Christ died for us."
(Romans 5:8 NIV)

There's no better feeling in the world than experiencing unconditional love. The feeling of safety, security, no judgment, no condemnation—just peace. That's what our Heavenly Father offers us. That's why He died for us—so we could be free from the burden of guilt, shame, and sin. God loved us so much that He died for us.

Yet we still live in bondage. It's like being given a gift, but we never unwrap the package to see what's inside. Or like having an electric fan on a scorching hot day, but never plugging it in. There's no need for us to feel broken and bound, when we've been set free. There's no need to stuff our feelings with food, when God always provides a way of escape. There's no need to feel hopeless, when God is our hope.

Take some time today to truly reflect on what Jesus died to give you. Purpose in your heart to be a reflection of His love toward you. Rest in the truth that He will never leave you nor forsake you, even when you mess up. Receive His grace today. He loves you with an everlasting love.

Today's Love Challenge

God loved us enough to die for us. What an affront to God when we fail to love and appreciate ourselves. For today's challenge, put on your favorite outfit. Take some time to care for yourself and exude the confidence that should come with knowing that God thought you were worth dying for. Journal your experience or thoughts after completing this challenge.

_____

_____

_____

_____

_____

Additional Study Scripture

"Let us then with confidence draw near to the throne of grace, that we may receive mercy and find grace to help in time of need."
(Hebrews 4:16 ESV)

"So that you may be sons of your Father who is in heaven. For he makes his sun rise on the evil and on the good, and sends rain on the just and on the unjust."
(Matthew 5:45 ESV)

1. Reflect on the depth of God's love for you. Allow the scripture to draw you closer to Him and journal your thoughts.

_____

_____

_____

_____

_____

_____

2. What keeps you from truly experiencing the depth of His love? Write them down and then place them at His feet.

_____

_____

_____

_____

_____

_____

3. Let God know that you want to experience the full depth and magnitude of His love for you.

_____

_____

_____

_____

_____

_____

_____

Today's Prayer

Dear Jesus, thank You so much that You didn't wait for me to get my act together before You loved me! It took me a while to realize it, God, but all I ever wanted was for someone to truly see me, truly know me, and then promise to never leave me. I tried many ways to earn love and fill that place on my own, and tried to get a lot of people to do it for me. I am so very sorry that I didn't truly grasp what You did for me and that I took You for granted. Thank You for the gift of your unconditional love and the priceless gift of Your ultimate sacrifice in the form of Jesus Christ. I receive this with thanks and praise. In Jesus' Name, Amen.

Day 7

God Rejoices Over You

Scripture Reflection

> *"The LORD your God is in your midst, a mighty*
> *one who will save; he will rejoice over you with*
> *gladness; he will quiet you by his love; he will exult*
> *over you with loud singing."*
> (Zephaniah 3:17 ESV)

Sometimes it's nice to have someone fawn over us—to tell us how special and wonderful we are, and to quiet our anxious spirit when we get all worked up. Many of us search high and low for that special someone. When we do, we put expectations on others that they can never possibly fulfill, and in the end we're always left feeling disappointed and frustrated.

We were never meant to go to others to fulfill needs that only God can fill. We were never meant to turn to food to fill the void, the hurt, the pain, and the unmet expectations. People and food might provide a temporary fix, but in the end it only creates a greater need. No food and no person can ever come close to meeting your unmet needs.

Yet such a person exists, and his name is Jesus. The scripture reminds us that He is always present, so we never have to feel alone or lonely. We can feel peace and joy because He will always save us (especially from ourselves). We can feel peace and joy because He will quiet our anxious spirit, fulfill our deepest craving and desires, and we can feel joy because He rejoices over us. Imagine having our own cheering section constantly encouraging us.

Today's Love Challenge

Take time today to receive that love that God so freely gives us. Write "I LOVE YOU" 10 times. If you feel like it, take some time and decorate the page.

Additional Study Scripture

*"For as a young man marries a young woman,
so shall your sons marry you, and as the
bridegroom rejoices over the bride, so shall
your God rejoice over you."*
(Isaiah 62:5 ESV)

"Jerusalem, Jerusalem, you who kill the prophets and stone those sent to you, how often I have longed to gather your children together, as a hen gathers her chicks under her wings, and you were not willing."
(Matt 23:27 NIV)

1. Reflect on the picture of Jesus rejoicing over you and quieting you with His love. How does that make you feel? (Zephaniah 3:17)

_____

_____

_____

_____

_____

2. Picture Jesus sitting with you right now. What is He saying to you? What are you saying to Him?

_____

_____

_____

_____

_____

3. Where have you been trying to find satisfaction other than from our God? Repent and let God know that you trust Him to meet all your needs.

_____

_____

_____

_____

_____

_____

_____

Today's Prayer

Lord Jesus, when I thought it was all about me it was easy to look at my faults and failures as things that made me less lovable. I tried to conceal and camouflage them as best I could because I needed love so badly. But God, now that I see that it's all about You and not about me I am free to be me! Set me free from comparisons, competition, people-pleasing, striving, lying, and hiding. I'm free in You, Jesus. Thank You! Help me to receive Your love fully, and to let it overflow onto all those around me. In Jesus' precious Name, Amen.

Day 8

But for the Grace of God!

Scripture Reflection

> *"But God, being rich in mercy, because of the great*
> *love with which he loved us, even when we were*
> *dead in our trespasses, made us alive together with*
> *Christ—by grace you have been saved."*
> (Ephesians 2:4-5 ESV)

I would have given into depression – **BUT GOD!**

I would have continued to be a slave to sin – **BUT GOD!**

I would have continued to suffer in silence and slowly continue to die inside – **BUT GOD!**

I would have continued to rebel against my own success, against my calling, and against who He called me to be – **BUT GOD!**

These two words could possibly be the two most welcome and powerful words in our vocabulary if we allow them to saturate our being. God loves us so much that He chose to save us despite ourselves. And despite our uncanny knack of trying to control every situation and choose our way instead of His.

As your feelings of anxiety, being overwhelmed, and frustration begin to creep in, pause for a moment and say, "But God."

When things don't turn out as planned, pause for a moment and say, "But God."

As you break your eating boundaries and want to beat up on yourself, pause for a moment and say, "But God."

As your family members start to grate on your last nerve, pause for a moment and say, "But God."

As you are saddened by all the injustice and chaos you see in the world, pause for a moment and say, "But God."

God loves us too much to ever leave us alone. His grace and His mercy are with us in every situation and every circumstance that we experience.

Today's Love Challenge

Write down a positive memory from the past that you remember was 'but for the grace of God'.

_____

_____

_____

_____

_____

_____

_____

Additional Study Scripture

"But he said to me, 'My grace is sufficient for you, for my power is made perfect in weakness.' Therefore, I will boast all the more gladly of my weaknesses, so that the power of Christ may rest upon me."
(2 Corinthians 12:9 ESV)

"I have been crucified with Christ and I no longer live, but Christ lives in me. The life I now live in the body, I live by faith in the Son of God, who loved me and gave himself for me."
(Galatians 2:20 NIV)

1. Reflect on the grace that God supplies you with each day. How does this make you feel?

_____

_____

_____

_____

2. Where do you need God's grace in your life today? It's available to you if you simply ask Him.

---

3. Ask the Holy Spirit to give you fresh insight into how and when you move away from God's grace and into 'works-based' living. Let Him lovingly keep guiding you back to grace.

Today's Prayer

Heavenly Father, I am astounded by Your power. You make the impossible possible. You make beauty from ashes. You bring to life the dead. So help me, when I feel the weight of the world beginning to cloud my vision, to say, "The world may be broken, but God, You are in control!" "My family may be difficult, but You give me the power to choose love." "I may feel tired, but You give me rest." Help me, Lord, when judgment and criticism come across my mind to remember that, but for the grace of God, there go I. In Jesus' Name, Amen.

Day 9

Unselfish Love

Scripture Reflection

> *"For God so loved the world, that he gave his only*
> *Son, that whoever believes in him should not perish*
> *but have eternal life."*
> (John 3:16 ESV)

It seems impossible for me to fathom a love so great that it would sacrifice everything for another.

My version of love pales in comparison to the depth of love that Jesus so freely gave you and me. My version of love is based on what I can feel, taste, or touch. It's hard for me to comprehend someone willing to die for me.

Because our 'human' version of love is so limited, instead of embracing this depth of love we waste precious time looking for love in all the wrong places. We look for love in the approval of others, we search for it in things that never satisfy us and we strive to reach higher in our accomplishments, believing that eventually we can 'feel it'.

But nothing will ever compare to the immeasurable love that God lavishes on us. He sacrificed His life so that you and I could live. Just think about that for a minute—you were worth dying for!

When we search for love in possessions, gifts, food, status or even social events, remember that the powerful act of love that God demonstrated to us on the cross is still available to us now.

Rest in the unselfish love of God today. Allow the truth of His ultimate sacrifice and relentless pursuit of you to calm your worried and anxious heart and racing mind.

Today's Love Challenge

In your journal, or on a sticky note, write this out: "I am loved lavishly by God."

Additional Study Scripture

"For your steadfast love is before my eyes,
and I walk in your faithfulness."
(Psalm 26:3 ESV)

"But God shows his love for us in that while we were
still sinners, Christ died for us."
(Romans 5:8 ESV)

"No, in all these things we are more than conquerors
through him who loved us. For I am sure that
neither death nor life, nor angels nor rulers, nor
things present nor things to come, nor powers, nor
height nor depth, nor anything else in all creation,
will be able to separate us from the love of God in
Christ Jesus our Lord."
(Romans 8:37-39 ESV)

1. Reflect on the unselfishness of God's love for you.

_____

_____

_____

_____

_____

_____

2. In what ways could you open your heart to the Father to teach you how to receive His love?

_____

_____

_____

_____

_____

_____

_____

_____

_____

_____

Today's Prayer

Dear Sweet Jesus, the truth about who You are and how You love me is too great for my mind to grasp. Sometimes I confess that I even doubt Your unconditional love to be true when I get trapped at looking at myself rather than keeping my eyes on You. I'm so sorry about that. Help me to remember the unconditional, sacrificial, heart-changing love You have for me and for others, and help me and them experience it deeply. I ask this in Jesus' Name. Amen.

Day 10

How He Loves Us

Scripture Reflection

> *"I have been crucified with Christ. It is no longer I*
> *who live, but Christ who lives in me. And the life I*
> *now live in the flesh I live by faith in the Son of God*
> *who loved me and gave himself for me."*
> (Galatians 2:20 NIV)

The Bible tells us clearly that we have been crucified with Christ, yet most of us live with the guilt and shame of our past every day. We live as if Christ's death is just something we read about, but has no direct impact on our lives or on how we see ourselves.

What if, effective immediately, you begin to live your life as if Christ truly lives in you? What if, when you looked in the mirror, you did not see your sin, your past, your mistakes, or your flaws?

What if you saw yourself the way God sees you? Would that have you walk with a bit more confidence? Would you worry less? Would you smile more? Would you care less about what people thought of you and more about how you could be a blessing to them?

Take time today to reflect on what God has done for you and begin to 'act as if' His death gave you a new life. Why? Because it's true!!!

Today's Love Challenge

Look at yourself in the mirror. Say to yourself what God says to you when He sees you. Use a verse or say whatever comes to your mind as you think of how much He loves you. Journal your experience or thoughts after completing this challenge.

_____

_____

_____

_____

_____

_____

_____

_____

_____

Additional Study Scripture

*"For sin will have no dominion over you, since you
are not under law but under grace."*
(Romans 6:14 ESV)

*"I, therefore, a prisoner for the Lord, urge you to walk
in a manner worthy of the calling to which you have
been called, with all humility and gentleness, with
patience, bearing with one another in love, eager to
maintain the unity of the Spirit in the bond of peace."*
(Ephesians 4:1-3 ESV)

*"Now to him who is able to do far more abundantly
than all that we ask or think, according to the power
at work within us, to him be glory in the church and
in Christ Jesus throughout all generations, forever
and ever. Amen."*
(Ephesians 3:20-21 ESV)

1. Meditate on the grace, power, and authority you have as a result of Christ's love for you.

_____

_____

_____

_____

_____

2. Take some time today to experience God's love, grace, and presence. Journal your experience.

_____

_____

_____

_____

_____

_____

_____

3. How can you walk in a manner worthy of your calling?

_____

_____

_____

_____

_____

_____

_____

Today's Prayer

Holy Father, Oh, how You love us! We are so thankful that when You look at us You don't see our sin. You don't see our blemishes, shortcomings, or imperfections. Because of the beautiful sacrifice of Your only Son, Jesus, You see His perfection imputed on us. Give me Your eyes to look upon myself and to look upon others, and let me see as You see, with the eyes of pure love. Please inspire my mind with creative reminders of Your grace, mercy, and unconditional love, so that when I do find an imperfection my mind quickly rejects that idea and my heart is filled with compassion and love. I pray this in Jesus' Name. Amen.

Day 11

Alive in Him

Scripture Reflection

*"But God, being rich in mercy, because of the great
love with which he loved us, even when we were
dead in our trespasses, made us alive together with
Christ—by grace you have been saved."*
(Ephesians 2:4-5 NIV)

Only God can bring life out of spiritual death. Only He can
bring light into darkness, and only He can make crooked paths
straight.

The Bible is replete with story after story of God's mercy
towards his people—Genesis 19:16, Philippians 2:27, Genesis
39:1-4, 1 Timothy 1:13, Luke 7:11-15, Daniel 2:9, to highlight
just a few.

Yet, despite these testimonies, we act as if we're still dead
in our trespasses. We still feel like our burdens are ours to carry
by ourselves. The Word says that He made us alive together with
Christ. Do you hear that?

1. You're alive, no longer dead in your trespasses.

2. Together with Christ—you don't have to do it on your own. It's a partnership—a relationship!

Declare that the dark areas of your life will shine bright with the love of the Lord.

Confess that the dead areas of your life will be resurrected, in the matchless Name of Jesus.

As you continually evaluate your life, remember God's perfect love. Life is not about mistakes, failures, or struggles, but about the God who loves us through it all.

Today's Love Challenge

Thank God for His precious gift of bringing you out of darkness and into His marvelous light. Thank Him for His great love for you. Let Him know how much you appreciate every aspect of your life, including the challenging areas. Journal your experience or thoughts after completing this challenge.

_____

_____

_____

_____

_____

Additional Study Scripture

"The steadfast love of the Lord never ceases;
his mercies never come to an end; they are new
every morning; great is your faithfulness."
(Lamentations 3:22-23 ESV)

"Bless the Lord, O my soul, and forget not all his
benefits, who forgives all your iniquity, who heals
all your diseases, who redeems your life from the pit,
who crowns you with steadfast love and mercy."
(Psalm 103:2-4 ESV)

1. Meditate on the steadfast love of the Lord. What does it mean to you?

_____

_____

_____

_____

2. Reflect on God's mercy in the following scriptures: Genesis 19:16, Philippians 2:27, Genesis 39:1-4, 1 Timothy 1:13, Luke 7:11-15, Daniel 2:9. How do they encourage you to walk in His mercy instead of in the weight of your sins?

_____

_____

_____

3. Think about your weight loss journey. How can it reflect Christ being alive in you?

_____

_____

_____

_____

_____

_____

_____

Today's Prayer

Dear Lord Jesus, I thank You that I get to be in a relationship with God the Father through You! That is the best gift ever!! I can see that I sometimes don't act as if You've already paid the penalty for my sins and died in my stead for each one of them. Would You forgive me and heal me of this rebellion against Your love? I want to love you back with a love as fervent as the one You have for me! God, I would be nothing without Your great love, and I simply thank You for loving me. Help me to live my life dead to sin and alive with You today and every day! In Jesus' Name, Amen.

Day 12

God's Unconditional Love

Scripture Reflection

"God shows his love for us in that while we were still sinners, Christ died for us."
(Romans 5:8 NIV)

God's unconditional love is the foundation of everything we do.

He does not love us sometimes. He doesn't love us anymore when we're doing the right thing, when we go to church, or when we're reading the Bible. He doesn't love us any less when we sin or break our boundaries. His love for us never changes.

So why do we sometimes go to Him and sometimes we hide from Him? It's not because He changes, it's because we feel shame from our sin. But if you truly want to experience the full depth of God's love for you, come and experience Him in all seasons and times of your life—when you feel close to Him, and especially when you've sinned.

Purpose to let Him into every part of your day and your life. Give Him your past, your present, and your future. Thank

Him when you eat within your boundaries, and call on Him when you break them. Give Him your schedule and ask Him to give you balance and order. Nothing you do or say will change the way that He feels about you.

Give Him this day. It will look a lot different when He is the driving force in it.

Purpose in your heart to live out of a revelation of God's unconditional love for you rather than living a fear-based relationship with Him. Remember, God loves you regardless of your weaknesses and failures.

Today's Love Challenge

Walk with confidence knowing that Christ died so that you could live—no shame, no guilt, no condemnation. Choose your favorite outfit today and wear it with confidence, fully saturating yourself in the truth that you are lavishly loved by God. Journal your experience or thoughts after completing this challenge.

Additional Study Scripture

"But if anyone loves God, he is known by God."
(1 Corinthians 8:3 ESV)

"No, in all these things we are more than conquerors through him who loved us. For I am sure that neither death nor life, nor angels nor rulers, nor things present nor things to come, nor powers, nor height nor depth, nor anything else in all creation, will be able to separate us from the love of God in Christ Jesus our Lord."
(Romans 8:37-39 ESV)

"Therefore, there is now no condemnation for those who are in Christ Jesus."
(Romans 8:1 ESV)

1. Reflect on God's unconditional love for you. Think about what that means to you.

_____

_____

_____

_____

_____

_____

2. If you truly believed that God's love is unconditional, how would that change the way you live?

_____

_____

_____

_____

_____

_____

3. Take time to receive God's unconditional love. With each breath, feel yourself receiving it within every cell of your body.

_____

_____

_____

_____

_____

_____

Today's Prayer

God, I am astounded that You can love me the way you do. The fact that there isn't anything I could do to make You love me more and not a single thing I could do to make You love me less than You do right now is mind-blowing!! Lord, I'm asking You for a heart-deep revelation of this love that is so hard for our finite human minds to even consider possible. Today, I give You my burdens, sins, joys, struggles, and failures. And in exchange I receive your boundless, total, and unconditional love into the depths of my heart. You are amazing, and I love You, Jesus. Amen.

Day 13

A Model of Love

Scripture Reflection

*"See what kind of love the Father has given to us,
that we should be called children of God; and so we
are. The reason why the world does not know us is
that it did not know him."*
(1 John 3:1 ESV)

As a recovering people-pleaser, I wasted far too many years worrying about what other people thought of me. I tried and tried to win the approval of others, but it only left me exhausted and disappointed. I realized that wanting to please others is not about others at all. It's all about me and my need to be needed.

God shows us in His Word that the foundation for loving others must come from Him, who is love. I'm learning that if I'm not plugged in to His love and grace, then my love for others will continue to be selfish and fear-based—nothing like the kind of love He has given to us.

For our faith to work, we must commit to loving one another as Christ has loved us. This requires constantly practicing selfless acts of mercy, grace, love, and respect. It requires putting our personal fears and limiting beliefs aside, and making a sacrificial commitment to love others as God loves us.

It's always difficult dealing with challenging family members—after all, they know our triggers and weaknesses better than anyone. Relationships can be messy, yet God commands us to love others. The more we can demonstrate Christ's love to others, the more we can open ourselves to experience His love for us.

Today's Love Challenge

Spend a few minutes today and think about how your Father has loved you. Then, based on the overflow of love in your heart, intentionally do something kind for someone else. Journal your experience or thoughts after completing this challenge.

_____

_____

_____

_____

_____

_____

_____

Additional Study Scripture

> *"And above all these put on love, which binds every-*
> *thing together in perfect harmony. And let the peace*
> *of Christ rule in your hearts, to which indeed you*
> *were called in one body."*
> (Colossians 3:14-15 ESV)

> *"Love one another with brotherly affection.*
> *Outdo one another in showing honor."*
> (Romans 12:10 ESV)

1. Reflect on what you often do for others. Do you do it out of Christ's love for you, or are there often other motivations?

_____

_____

_____

_____

_____

2. How can you show brotherly affection to others?

_____

_____

_____

_____

3. Imagine yourself as an open conduit for love. As you receive Christ's love, you pass it on to others. How does it feel being used by God in such a way?

_____

_____

_____

_____

_____

_____

_____

_____

Today's Prayer

Dearest God, You've shown us the kind of love that comes from having a "You-first" heart, rather than a "me-first" one. I need You to change my heart, please. I want to obey Your command to love others, and I admit that it is hard to love at times. Your model of love says that we don't love only when we feel like it—we do it because You loved us first. Lord, please point out any places inside of me where I feel unlovable and come straight into them. I welcome You. Set me free to love, Jesus, and I thank You in advance for that freedom. In Jesus' Name, Amen.

Day 14

Love is a Verb

Scripture Reflection

> *"Beloved, let us love one another, for love is from
> God, and whoever loves has been born of God and
> knows God. Anyone who does not love does not know
> God, because God is love."*
> (1 John 4:7–8 NIV)

The disciple John was the foremost writer about the topic of love in the Bible. Much of his teaching and writings focus on love being an action instead of a feeling.

We want to 'feel' love, but John shows us how God doesn't just give a feeling of love. He demonstrates His love to us through action.

> *"For God so loved the world that he gave his one
> and only Son."*
> (John 3:16 NIV)

> *"The Father loves the Son and has placed
> all things under his authority."*
> (John 3:35 NET)

"For the Father loves the Son and shows him
everything he does, and will show him greater deeds
than these, so that you will be amazed."
(John 5:20 NET)

There is no force more powerful than the love that our Heavenly Father has for us. His love corrects us, calms our anxious hearts, moves mountains out of our way, breaks strongholds, transforms us, and heals our brokenness. God is love, and His love is living and active. It's not simply a warm, fuzzy feeling that brings us temporary relief. God's love always displays an action, so let's follow His example.

Today's Love Challenge

Do something for yourself today to show your love for God. Offer Him a sacrifice, tell God you love Him, think of how you can be of service to someone in need, or volunteer your time on God's behalf. How can you be of service to someone? Journal your experience or thoughts after completing this challenge.

_____

_____

_____

_____

_____

_____

Additional Study Scripture

*"In this the love of God was made manifest among
us, that God sent his only Son into the world, so that
we might live through him. In this is love, not that we
have loved God but that he loved us and sent his Son
to be the propitiation for our sins."*
(1 John 4:9–10 ESV)

*"So we have come to know and to believe the love
that God has for us. God is love, and whoever abides
in love abides in God, and God abides in him."*
(1 John 4:16 ESV)

1. Reflect on how God shows His love for us through action.
What has He done for you?

_____

_____

_____

_____

2. What will you do to show God how much you love Him
and abide in Him?

_____

_____

_____

_____

3. Think of your weight loss journey. How can you demonstrate your love for God? What actions can you take?

_____

_____

_____

_____

_____

_____

_____

_____

_____

Today's Prayer

Thank You so much, God, that You're not asking me to wait until I FEEL like loving in order to love! I'm grateful that, since this is something You command of me, it means that it's something I can CHOOSE to do. Thank You that Your love is no temporary fix or fleeting feeling—it is a rock that I can stand on. It's a promise I can hold fast to; it's the salve that heals my weary soul. Help me to love out of a heart that yields to others as I act sacrificially—giving before receiving, understanding before explaining, and listening before speaking. In Jesus' Name, Amen.

Day 15

God Sings to You

Scripture Reflection

> *"The LORD your God is in your midst, a mighty*
> *one who will save; he will rejoice over you with*
> *gladness; he will quiet you by his love; he will exult*
> *over you with loud singing."*
> (Zephaniah 3:17 NIV)

It really is hard to fathom just how much God loves us.

I have felt an indescribable depth of love for my son. I remember when he was a baby and I would constantly sing songs to him to soothe him when he was crying. Or I would just sing to him to let him know how much I loved him.

I also remember my husband sending me love songs by popular artists. He is tone deaf but wanted to express his love for me in song. Listening to these songs warmed my heart and touched a special place in my spirit.

The Bible tells us that God does the same for us. It says that He will exult over us with loud singing. Can you imagine that? We sing songs of love to God, maybe during Sunday service, but have you ever imagined Him singing to us? This is how much joy and delight we give the Lord—that He breaks into song when He thinks of us!

Today, purpose to grasp the magnitude of the love and joy God has for you. I know His love for us is on a level that we can't imagine, but let's begin to experience His love by simply spending time with Him as He beckons us.

When you feel overwhelmed or stressed, think of God singing a love song to you!

Today's Love Challenge

Imagine God exulting over you with singing. Play one of your favorite songs and visualize your Heavenly Father singing this song to you. Journal your experience or thoughts after completing this challenge.

_____

_____

_____

_____

_____

_____

_____

Additional Study Scripture

"Just so, I tell you, there is joy before the angels
of God over one sinner who repents."
(Luke 15:10 ESV)

Meditate on Zephaniah 3:17. Highlight the specific verses that minister to you.

_____

_____

_____

_____

_____

As you think about God singing over you, allow the Holy Spirit to fill you with His joy and peace.

_____

_____

_____

_____

_____

Today's Prayer

God, I come before You now to simply be there at Your feet, curled up on Your lap, right there in Your arms. As I inhale, I breathe in the aroma of Your sweet love. And as I exhale I send out stress, fear, anxiety, and trouble from inside of me. Lord, as I stay with You I can start to sense Your compassion on me. I can feel it through Your touch, Your embrace, Your soft gaze on me. You delight over me, my Lord, and I welcome it. Sing Your Heavenly songs to my heart, Jesus. I now surrender fully to the magnificence of Your amazing grace and unfailing love. In Jesus' Name, Amen.

Day 16

Joy on the Journey

Scripture Reflection

> *"And God will wipe away every tear from their eyes;*
> *there shall be no more death, nor sorrow, nor crying.*
> *There shall be no more pain, for the former things*
> *have passed away."*
> (Revelation 21:4 NIV)

God's perspective on trials and hardship is very different from ours. We want it over as quickly as possible or, more accurately, we would rather not experience any hardships at all.

God sees the brokenness, difficulties and trials, and He celebrates. Not because He is merciless, but because He knows the end from the beginning. He knows that one day soon it will all be redeemed. He rejoices in the fact that, one day, *"he will wipe away every tear from their eyes, and death shall be no more, neither shall there be mourning, nor crying, nor pain anymore, for the former things have passed away"*. Imagine if we could see life from His perspective.

If we will be patient and trust God to redeem the trials and difficulties we experience in this life, we will begin to spend less time worrying and more time experiencing His peace. Joy is our portion and we can experience joy on our journey, even when things are not joyful.

Rest in His presence and search out the heart of our King. Experience the fullness of joy that comes from spending time with God during this holiday season and always.

Today's Love Challenge

Spend 10 minutes in silence focusing on what truly brings you joy. Write it down and then give thanks to God for all the joy He has given you.

_____

_____

_____

_____

_____

_____

_____

_____

_____

Additional Study Scripture

"Count it all joy, my brothers, when you meet trials of various kinds, for you know that the testing of your faith produces steadfastness. And let steadfastness have its full effect, that you may be perfect and complete, lacking in nothing."
(James 1:2-4 ESV)

"You make known to me the path of life; in your presence there is fullness of joy; at your right hand are pleasures forevermore."
(Psalm 16:11 ESV)

"You have put more joy in my heart than they have when their grain and wine abound."
(Psalm 4:7 ESV)

1. Reflect on trials and tribulations from God's perspective. How are they different from your perspective?

_____

_____

_____

_____

_____

_____

2. Think about your weight loss journey. How can you use the trials and difficulties as an opportunity to draw closer to God?

_____

_____

_____

_____

3. Imagine God wiping away your tears. Visualize Him there with you in the hard times. Find comfort in His presence.

_____

_____

_____

_____

Today's Prayer

Heavenly Father, thank You so much for the promise that You will wipe away every tear from our eyes; that there won't be any more pain, crying, or mourning. Lord, would You explore my heart and show me places where I'm not accepting Your sovereignty over my life, and show me how that is robbing me of my joy? I want to come into alignment with Your view, that You work all things together for my good and your glory! So even when it's hard to feel happy, Lord, I thank You that I get to have joy on the inside. In Jesus' Name, Amen.

Day 17

Rest in His Presence

Scripture Reflection

"Humble yourselves, therefore, under the mighty hand of God so that at the proper time he may exalt you, casting all your anxieties on him, because he cares for you."
(1 Peter 5:6-7 NIV)

Why do we continue to carry our burdens and worries, when God tells us it's not necessary? Because deep down inside we don't fully trust God. We don't truly believe that He can handle our messes better than we can. Or maybe we don't feel that we can go to God because we can't expect Him to get us out of a mess that we got ourselves into. Or could it be that we've struggled for so long that it's become our identity, and we feel like it's just who we are—a lifelong struggler (one who believes that life is supposed to be hard)?

Whatever category you find yourself in, realize that your current identity does not have to become your destiny. God truly cares for you, and will restore you in due season as you learn to trust Him. That's how much He loves you.

What will be required of you is humility—a letting go of the perfectionism, the need to control, and the need to feel like you must do it on your own. Besides, it's not working for you anyway, is it? Stop trying so hard and learn to rest in Him.

Let your life be marked by simplicity—by rest and by ease, instead of our default which is overwhelmed and complex. Trust that God will help you accomplish everything you need to do in a timely and productive manner, this and every other season of your life. Trust that He will give you the strength when you're feeling weak.

Today's Love Challenge

Go to bed 30 minutes earlier and love yourself by getting some more rest. As you go to sleep, thank God for loving you so richly, caring for you so deeply, and for ordering your steps. Journal your experience or thoughts after completing this challenge.

Additional Study Scripture

*"Come to me, all who labor and are heavy laden, and
I will give you rest. Take my yoke upon you, and learn
from me, for I am gentle and lowly in heart, and you
will find rest for your souls. For my yoke is easy,
and my burden is light."*
(Matthew 11:28–30 ESV)

*"Six days you shall work, but on the seventh day
you shall rest. In plowing time and in harvest you
shall rest."*
(Exodus 34:21 ESV)

1. Meditate on God's desire to have you cast your cares on Him. Allow the scripture to bring you peace.

_____

_____

_____

_____

_____

_____

_____

2. Think of the busyness of the season you're currently in. Where can you exchange complexity for simplicity and stress for ease?

_____

_____

_____

_____

3. Where are you trying to do things in your own strength on your weight loss journey? What will you turn over to God?

_____

_____

_____

_____

Today's Prayer

Dear God, thank You that You are the great I AM. That I have nothing to fear because You are with me. That I can come to You with all my burdens and truly rest. I can see that I've been stubbornly holding on to some things rather than releasing them to You. Lord, I'm sorry for this attitude and I ask You to forgive me and heal me. Help me to cease from striving and controlling and to allow myself to step into the ease of Your rest—right beside the peaceful, calm stream. I pray this in Jesus' Name. Amen.

Day 18

Amazing Love!

Scripture Reflection

> *"But you, O Lord, are a God merciful and gracious, slow to anger and abounding in steadfast love and faithfulness."*
> (Psalm 86:15 ESV)

When I read stories in the Bible I'm blown away by God's love, mercy, and compassion. For example, I can't believe that David could murder and commit adultery and be considered a man after God's own heart. I cringe when I think about the Israelites worshiping a golden calf 'after' Moses made a covenant with God. And don't even get me started with Paul—murdering Christians! That 'should' be unforgivable (at least to you and me).

But when God uses the word 'abounding', He wants us to understand that His love is not like how we view love. His love has no boundaries or limits. The resources of His love are not limited. His love is limitless, and His power is limitless.

God wants us to know that, regardless of what we've done or what circumstances we face—whether in a season of chaos and frustration, during this Christmas season or during a dark time of trial—God's love is our compass, our ever-present, inexhaustible source of strength.

As you continually slip up on your weight loss journey, know that God is not mad at you and He will never turn His back on you. Like David and Paul, He wants you to return to Him. He wants you to understand the depth of His compassionate heart.

We will never be able to understand the depth of God's love for us, and we may not feel that we deserve it, but that's the beauty of His love. It's beyond comprehension. May His amazing love enlighten you, challenge you, motivate you, and inspire you to draw close to Him.

Love Challenge

Instead of focusing on your faults, give yourself a pat on the back for something you've accomplished.

_____

_____

_____

_____

_____

_____

Additional Study Scripture

*"The Lord is merciful and gracious, slow to anger
and abounding in steadfast love."*
(Psalm 103:8 ESV)

*"Can a woman forget her nursing child, that she
should have no compassion on the son of her
womb? Even these may forget, yet I will not forget
you. Behold, I have engraved you on the palms of my
hands; your walls are continually before me."*
(Isaiah 49:15–16 ESV)

1. Meditate on God's abounding love for you. Journal your thoughts.

_____

_____

_____

_____

2. Ask the Holy Spirit to help you encounter and experience the depth of God's abounding love for you.

_____

_____

_____

_____

3. Reflect on a biblical character who confessed their sin and God forgave them. That's how abounding His love is towards you, too. Journal the similarities that come to mind.

_____

_____

_____

_____

_____

_____

_____

_____

Today's Prayer

Lord, Your love is amazing. It's awe-inspiring. It's astounding. It's incomprehensible to my finite, human mind. However, despite that, I'm willing to believe that You're real, that Your love is true, and that it's personally and intimately for me. Help me to bathe in that amazing love right now, Father, not because I've done something to deserve it, but because You've done everything so that I can have it. I pray that my sisters and I would each receive a brand-new revelation of how much You love us. In Jesus' Name, Amen.

Day 19

Seeking the Gift-Giver

Scripture Reflection

"For I know the plans I have for you," declares the
LORD. "Plans to prosper you and not to harm you,
plans to give you hope and a future."
(Jeremiah 29:11 NIV)

I've gotta admit, I spend a lot of time worrying about missing God. What if I miss His plan for my life? What if I take the wrong path? What if it wasn't God's voice I was hearing at all but the enemy's, trying to lead me away from God?

It's hard to admit, but when I really think about it I think my fear is because what I'm really seeking is the gift and not the Gift-Giver. My fear is because I may not get what I want. I want His will 'if' that makes my life more prosperous, joyous, and easy. And when I don't receive it, then I don't believe it was really God. What if God's will means giving up all my creature comforts and 'my' dreams and desires? Would I still go along with His plans?

As I grow in the Lord, I'm reminded that every good and beautiful dream we have in this life came from our good Father in the first place. God knows what's best for us. He knows us better than we know ourselves, and He will never lead us down the wrong path (like we sometimes do to ourselves).

God has given us gifts of wisdom and discernment to make the right choices. If we seek Him instead of what He can give us, we won't miss Him. God is not a moving target that we have to try to shoot like a game at a carnival. Once we've submitted to Him we don't have to be filled with worry, fretting about whether we made the right decision.

Yes, we might miss God sometimes, but let's remember that God is bigger than our mistakes and missteps. God knows the end from the beginning, and He promises to work all things out for our good as we seek Him (Romans 8:28).

Walk in the confidence and peace that God's plans are good and perfect. Receive His gift of peace, and that you will not miss Him or His will for your life if you continue to walk closely with Him. Let relationship with Him be your main goal.

Today's Love Challenge

Think of a decision that you need to make right now. Seek God and tell Him that you trust Him 100% with His perfect plan for your life. Then thank Him for an answer.

_____

_____

_____

_____

Additional Study Scripture

*"And we know [with great confidence] that God
[who is deeply concerned about us] causes all things
to work together [as a plan] for good for those who
love God, to those who are called according to His
plan and purpose."*
(Romans 8:28 AMP)

*"Until now you have asked nothing in my name. Ask,
and you will receive, that your joy may be full."*
(John 16:24 ESV)

*"But the fruit of the Spirit is love, joy, peace, patience,
kindness, goodness, faithfulness."*
(Galatians 5:22 ESV)

1. Reflect on God's heart to give you His best for you. What is He showing you?

_____

_____

_____

_____

_____

_____

2. How can you stop second-guessing God and trust His plans for you?

_____

_____

_____

_____

3. What are God's plans for your weight loss?

_____

_____

_____

_____

_____

Today's Prayer

Dear Lord, You are a good, good Father, and I love You so much! I come before You in Jesus' Name, honestly admitting that sometimes I'm seeking after stuff rather than Your face. You've told me to seek Your face and seek Your Kingdom, and I apologize for how much that must hurt Your heart when I just go to You with my hands open. Make me thirst more for Your living water and increase my hunger for Your Word each day. Make my heart's deepest desire be to know You better and to love You more. I seek more of You and less of me, Jesus. Amen.

Day 20
Overwhelming Victory with God

Scripture Reflection

> *"No, in all these things we are more than conquerors through him who loved us. For I am sure that neither death nor life, nor angels nor rulers, nor things present nor things to come, nor powers, nor height nor depth, nor anything else in all creation, will be able to separate us from the love of God in Christ Jesus our Lord."*
> (Romans 8:37–39 ESV)

Imagine that! Nothing can separate us from God's love. Absolutely nothing—no situation, no sin, no circumstance—because God's love encompasses everything. Think about the worst thing that you've done. You may be experiencing a lot of guilt, shame, and condemnation over it, but God does not love you any less as a result. He still sees you as His beloved child.

In the scripture above, Paul reminds us that we are MORE than conquerors through Him who loved us. To be "more than a conqueror" means we not only achieve victory, but we have an overwhelming victory. The outcome is even better than we could have anticipated.

Today and always, may the love of God keep you and sustain you in every situation with the knowledge that nothing in this world can ever separate you from God's love through our Lord and Savior Jesus Christ. Stand firm in your faith, because not only will you win but you will have an overwhelming victory.

Today's Love Challenge

Dare to do something bold. Step out in faith. It can be as subtle as wearing something you were too self-conscious to wear, have a conversation with someone you've been putting off, or risk sharing your faith with someone else if you've never done it before.

_____

_____

_____

_____

_____

_____

_____

_____

Additional Study Scripture

*"Where shall I go from your Spirit? Or where shall I
flee from your presence? If I ascend to heaven, you
are there! If I make my bed in Sheol, you are there!
If I take the wings of the morning and dwell in the
uttermost parts of the sea, even there your hand shall
lead me, and your right hand shall hold me. If I say,
'Surely the darkness shall cover me, and the light
about me be night,' even the darkness is not dark to
you; the night is bright as the day, for darkness is as
light with you."*
(Psalm 139:7–12 ESV)

*"The Lord will fight for you, and you have only to be
silent."*
(Exodus 14:14 ESV)

1. Meditate on the biblical truth that you are 'more than a conqueror'.

_____

_____

_____

_____

_____

_____

2. Think of an area of your life where you feel defeated. Apply Romans 8:37-39 to your situation.

_____

_____

_____

_____

3. Ask the Holy Spirit to give you a revelation of your overwhelming victory in your health and weight releasing journey.

_____

_____

_____

_____

Today's Prayer

Thank You, Lord, that this is not some by-the-skin-of-our-teeth victory You've won, but an OVERWHELMING victory You have secured for Your Kingdom and Your children! I pray that You would help me live with the deep inner-knowing that this victory has already been won and that there is absolutely nothing that can separate me from Your love. Thank You, Lord, that I get to stand firm in my faith and step out in it boldly because You love me. In Jesus' Name, Amen.

Day 21

In This is Love

Scripture Reflection

> *"In this the love of God was made manifest among us, that God sent his only Son into the world, so that we might live through him. In this is love, not that we have loved God but that he loved us and sent his Son to be the propitiation for our sins. Beloved, if God so loved us, we also ought to love one another."*
> (1 John 4:9–11 ESV)

What is love?

We use it in all sorts of contexts:

"I love ice cream."

"I love him."

"I love that show."

We can toss it around so much that we can lose the true impact and intensity of the word. And, sadly, since many of us have never come close to experiencing the depth of love that our Heavenly Father has for us, it's easy to think that the diluted forms we experience are the real thing. It's impossible to fathom the depth of love that our Daddy has for us because we've never experienced anything like it.

In the scripture above, the apostle John gets to the crux of love. He teaches us that God is love, and then goes on to tell us the depth of love God shows His children.

Here's what John shows us:

- God created us in His image – "In this is love."

- God cares for us in the midst of our sin – "In this is love."

- God sent His only Son to die for us on the cross – "In this is love."

Although we may never fully comprehend the depth of this love, I hope that this devotional has given you some insight into what love really means. This is just a taste of the magnitude of love that we can experience each day as we commune with our Heavenly Father.

Beloved, let's reach out and receive this incredible gift of love. It is the single most important thing we can do each day.

Open your heart to the reality of God's presence, love, and grace in your life—"In this is love."

Today's Love Challenge

Write a love letter to God, thanking Him for loving you so completely. Pour out your heart to Him in your letter.

_____

_____

_____

_____

_____

_____

_____

_____

Additional Study Scripture

*"For God so loved the world, that he gave his only
Son, that whoever believes in him should not perish
but have eternal life."*
(John 3:16 ESV)

*"A new commandment I give to you, that you love
one another: just as I have loved you, you also are to
love one another."*
(John 13:34 ESV)

1. Reflect on the depth of God's love for you. What is the Holy Spirit showing you?

_____

_____

_____

_____

_____

_____

2. Think of all the ways you don't love yourself and contrast it with how much God loves you. Repent for not loving yourself as much as He loves you.

_____

_____

_____

_____

_____

_____

3. How can you use your weight loss journey to get a fresh revelation of the depth of God's love for you?

_____

_____

_____

_____

_____

_____

_____

Today's Prayer

Dear Jesus, today I reach out my arms to You wide and say, "Yes to Your love! Yes, to Your forgiveness! Yes, to Your grace!" I say, "YES to You, my Heavenly Father!" As I prepare my heart to write a love letter to You, I ask Your forgiveness for all the times I didn't believe that You loved me. You've only asked for my heart, and sometimes I wasn't willing to give it to You. I'm so sorry. Thank You for hearing my prayer, granting me forgiveness, blessing me with Your presence, and never, ever forsaking me! I can't thank You enough for showing me what love really is. In Jesus' Name, Amen.

Day 22

My Exceeding Joy

Scripture Reflection

"To him who is able to keep you from stumbling and
to present you before his glorious presence without
fault and with great joy."
(Jude 1:24 NIV)

We have much reason to celebrate and be joyful for.

Joy is not something that happens to you. It's something that you cultivate. When you ground your life in the truth of our Savior, joy is everywhere.

As you celebrate milestones in your life, purpose in your heart to be filled with joy. Not because of the milestones them-selves but because of God's love for you.

You may be wondering how can you begin to experience this joy.

Choose to center your life around who Jesus is. Choose to surrender your thoughts, your feelings, your actions, your hab-its, and even your fears to God's unwavering love. As the world continually pulls you out of alignment and distracts you with frivolous and mundane things, continue to choose joy.

It's your gift from your Heavenly Father today and always. Everything you need to live a life of joy has been provided for you in the heart of God because He loves you so much.

May your life be filled with exceeding joy as we celebrate our Lord and Savior, Jesus Christ.

Today's Love Challenge

Make a list of all the reasons you are joyful.

_____

_____

_____

_____

_____

_____

_____

_____

Additional Study Scripture

"For his anger is but for a moment, and his favor is for a lifetime. Weeping may tarry for the night, but joy comes with the morning."
(Psalm 30:5)

"You make known to me the path of life; in your presence there is fullness of joy; at your right hand are pleasures forevermore."
(Psalm 16:11)

1. Reflect on God's desire to fill you with exceeding joy.

_____

_____

_____

_____

_____

2. Where in your life do you need joy?

_____

_____

_____

_____

_____

3. How can find joy on your weight loss journey?

Today's Prayer

Lord, I thank You for this devotional. It has blessed me immeasurably. Thank You for the tidings of great joy that You've restored in me. Thank You for Jesus and the joy and peace that floods my heart when I think of this ultimate sacrifice. Lord, we know that only in Him can true joy be found. As we celebrate life, remind me that You are the reason why I celebrate and that receiving Your love is the ultimate gift! I pray that true joy would come into the world this season and that others who don't know You will find joy, hope, and peace in You. All this I ask in Jesus' Name. Amen!

THANK YOU

Thank you for being motivated, courageous, inquisitive and committed to go deeper in your health journey and uncover the missing piece- Christ! I pray that these principles have been as much of a blessing to you as they have been for me and the hundreds of thousands of women around the world that have experienced what it means to include God in their health and weight-releasing journey.

If you've been blessed by this book, then please don't keep it a secret!

There are millions of women who need to hear this message. Please take a moment to leave an honest book review so more people can discover this book as well.

This book has laid out a great foundation for you, but there's so much more for you to discover. Please keep in touch with me so that you can stay in this conversation and continue to make your health a priority--God's Way. I'll send you a free copy of my '3 Steps to Overcoming Emotional Eating' guide, and a discount for an online version of this devotion, when you enroll for my weekly emails on successful weight loss, God's way.

lovegodloseweightbonus.com

Leader's Guide

"Therefore go and make disciples of all nations,
baptizing them in the name of the Father and of the
Son and of the Holy Spirit, and teaching them to obey
everything I have commanded you. And surely I am
with you always, to the very end of the age."
(Matt 19:20)

Thank you for answering the call to lead a group through the 21-day challenge. Coming together as a group holds you accountable and provides an opportunity to develop consistency within your faith. The best way to learn is to teach. We believe that as you lead others, you will also continue to grow in the Lord.

Healthy by Design ignites and mobilizes leaders who want to use their spiritual gifts and skills so that others can be transformed by the truth of God's Word.

Know that when you say 'yes' to minister to others, you are changing and affecting not only their lives but also the lives of everyone they come in contact with. You will find that, as a leader, you will feel more connected with the devotionals as you take on a sense of ownership and responsibility and want to support your small group as much as possible.

You have the option of leading the 21-day challenge online or in an in-person group. As a leader, you must register your courses with us. Please register your group here:

https://www.cathymorenzie.com/become-a-bible-study-leader/

The 21-day challenge/devotional works best when participants work independently and follow up their independent study with leader-led small-group interaction either in person or virtually. As the group leader, your responsibility is to facilitate discussion and conversation and make sure that everyone gets the most out of the devotionals. You are not responsible for having all the answers to people's questions or reteaching the content. That's what the devotional is for.

Your role is to guide the experience, encourage your group to go deeper into God's Word, cultivate an atmosphere of learning and growth amongst a body of believers, and answer any questions that the group may have.

Tips to get the most from the Small Groups Sessions

1. **It's about God.** Although we use biblical principles to guide us on how to address strongholds in our lives, at the end of the day remember that it's always about God. Your role as a leader is to always point everyone to the cross.

2. **Partner up.** Have your group choose an accountability partner to go through the devotional with. It's always more encouraging when you can connect with

someone on a regular basis in addition to when you meet as a group.

3. **Keep a journal.** Encourage your group to use a supplemental journal. They can choose from an online journal like Penzu (penzu.com) or use old-school pen and paper. Either way, taking time to record your thoughts, feelings, inspirations, and directives from the Holy Spirit is a great way to maximize the experience.

4. **Be consistent.** Meet at the same time and location each week. This will help the group to organize their time and their schedules. Try to select a time that works best for everyone.

5. **Plan ahead.** Take time prior to the weekly study to think about how you will present the material. Think about a story or example that would add to the material. Think about the most effective way to make use of the time.

6. **Keep it intimate.** Keep the small group small. I suggest a maximum of 12-15 people. This will create a more relaxed and transparent atmosphere so that people will feel safe to speak.

7. **Be transparent.** You can set the tone for the group by sharing your story. This will help people to feel safe and establish trust with them. When you speak, give personal examples and avoid phrases like 'some people' and 'Christians'.

8. **Be professional.** Always start and end the sessions on time. Communicate clearly if you see that you will be going over-time. Apologize and let them know how much you respect their time.

9. **Bring lots of energy.** Let your passion for studying God's Word be evident. Remember that your energy level will set the tone for the entire group, so bring it!

10. **Pray.** It might sound obvious, but make sure that prayer is an intricate part of the entire process. Pray at the beginning and end of every session. Feel free to call on others to lead the prayers. During the session, you can have one person pray for the entire group— have one person open and another close—ask for requests, or select someone. You can also encourage the group to pray for one another. Lastly, don't forget to pray during the time leading up to the session.

11. **Keep it simple.** If the sessions get too complicated, people will find reasons not to attend. If you plan to serve snacks, keep it simple and nutritious. Don't plan weekly potlucks that will require the group members to do too much work.

12. **Be creative.** Feel free to add music, props, or anything that you feel will add to the environment and facilitate learning.

13. **Be comfortable.** Make sure there is adequate comfortable seating for everyone. Check the temperature in the room. Alert everyone as to where the bathrooms are located.

Preliminary Preparation

- Pray and seek the Holy Spirit on whether you should participate in this devotional.

- Determine with your group how long you will meet each week, so you can plan your time accordingly. Most groups like to meet from 1-2 hours.

- Promote the Bible study through community announcements, social media, in your church bulletin, or simply call a few of your friends.

- Send out an email to a list or send a message on social media announcing the upcoming study.

- Prior to the first meeting, make sure that everyone purchases a copy of the devotional. Include a link where they can buy it.

- Have the group read Day 1 and be prepared to share their responses.

Suggested Group Plan

Because *Love God, Lose Weight* is an independent devotional, the group discussion will incorporate a series of small discussions within the greater discussion. Feel free to customize the design to fit the needs of your group. The suggested plan is for a four-week session. Following is the breakdown.

A Four-Week Session Plan

Session 1

1. Welcome everyone to the session and open with prayer.

2. Share a bit about yourself. Then go around the room and have everyone introduce themselves. Have each person share what their Christmas season is like. What are the challenges and stresses they face?

3. Give an overview of the devotional and a brief over-view of the *Love God, Lose Weight* Program.

4. Housekeeping Items:

- format for the session

- confirm dates and times

- where bathrooms are

- rules for sharing

- commitment to confidentiality

- attendance each week

- snacks (have volunteers provide)

5. Offer suggestions to get the most out of the study. Discuss the weekly love challenge and encourage the group to complete them instead of just reading them.

6. Stress the importance of trust and transparency.

7. Instruct the group to complete the six days before the next session. Encourage them to carve out some time each day to complete the devotions.

8. Review the Day 1 devotion and ask the group to share their responses.

Suggested Discussion Starters:

• What did you think about the analogy of the different types of flowers judging themselves? Did it make you think about how you compare yourself to others?

• What does it mean to you to be created in God's image?

• What would your life look like if you truly lived out that truth?

9. Have the group read Days 2-7 for next week's session.

10. Close the session in prayer.

Session 2

1. Welcome the group.

2. Start with an opening prayer.

3. Ask the group what insights/breakthroughs/testimonials they encountered as a result of what the Holy Spirit has been showing them.

Suggested Discussion Starters (from Days 2-7):

- Reflect on God's steadfast love in your life. Think of all the ways He has loved you.

- What is stealing your peace?

- Think about all the things you take for granted. Now give thanks to God for all of them. Does it change your perspective?

- What keeps you from truly experiencing the depth of God's love?

- Picture Jesus sitting with you right now. What is He saying to you? What are you saying to Him?

- Ask the group which of the devotions in Week 1 were most impactful for them.

4. Make a closing remark or statement to tie in the entire conversation.

5. Have the group read Days 8–14 for next week's session.

6. End with a closing prayer.

Session 3

1. Welcome the group.

2. Start with an opening prayer.

3. Ask the group what insights/breakthroughs/testimonials they encountered as a result of what the Holy Spirit has been showing them.

Suggested Discussion Starters (from Days 8–14):

- Where do you need God's grace in your life today?

- In what ways could you open your heart and accept His gift of love?

- Think of the grace, power, and love you possess as a result of God's love for you.

- How can you walk in a manner worthy of your calling?

- Think about your weight loss journey. How can it reflect Christ being alive in you?

- If you truly believed that God's love is unconditional, how would that change the way you live?

- What will you do to show God how much you love Him and abide in Him?

4. Have the group read Days 15-21 for next week's session.

5. End with a closing prayer.

Session 4

Think about how you will make the final session memorable. Maybe end with a nutritious meal, exchange written gifts, or organize something small that symbolizes God's love.

1. Welcome the group.

2. Start with an opening prayer.

3. Ask the group what insights/breakthroughs/tes-
   timonials they encountered as a result of what the
   Holy Spirit has been showing them.

Suggested Discussion Starters (from Days 15-21):

- Think about your weight loss journey. How can you
  use the trials and difficulties as an opportunity to
  draw closer to God?

- Think of the busyness of the season. Where can you
  exchange complexity for simplicity and stress for
  ease?

- Reflect on biblical characters who confessed their
  sins and God forgave them. How do you feel about
  that?

- How can you stop second-guessing God and trust
  His plans for you?

- Think of all the ways you don't love yourself and
  contrast it with how much God loves you.

- Where are you trying to do things in your own
  strength on your weight loss journey? What will you
  turn over to God?

4. Wrap up the session with closing words/thoughts.

5. End the session with a closing prayer.

Thank you again for taking the time to lead your group. You
are making a difference in the lives of others and having an impact on the Kingdom of God.

Other Healthy by Design Offerings

Healthy by Design (healthybydesignprogram.com) equips women to rely on God as their strength so they can live in freedom, joy, and peace. At the end of the day, that's what we really want. Let's be honest, if you never achieved that mythical, illusive number on the scale, but were fully able to live a life of freedom, joy, and peace, would that be enough? I know for me the answer is a resounding 'YES!!!'

We provide a multidimensional approach to releasing weight. It encompasses the whole person—spiritual, psychological, mental, nutritional, physical, and even hormonal! We believe that you must address the whole person—body, soul, and spirit. If you're looking for a program that just tells you what to eat and what exercises to do, this ain't it.

This program has helped thousands of women break free from all the roadblocks that have been hindering their weight loss success while discovering their identity in Christ.

Healthy by Design offers a variety of free and paid courses and programs. They include the following:

A YouVersion Bible Study

A free basic introduction to Step 1 of the WLGW program. To learn more, go to:

https://my.bible.com/reading-plans/4593-weight-loss-gods-way.com

Or from the YouVersion Bible App, click the bottom center, 'check-mark' button to open devotions, and search for 'Weight Loss God's Way or our other free devotionals:

Rest, Restore, and Rejuvenate

Praying for Your Health

The Weight Loss, God's Way Newsletter

Join the free *Weight Loss, God's Way* community and receive weekly posts designed to help you align your weight loss with God's Word. You'll also receive our Love Letters from God free download. To join the newsletter, sign up at:

lovegodloseweightbonus.com

The Membership Program

A done-for-you, step-by-step guide to the entire program. Dozens of bonus tools like group coaching calls, forums, and accountability groups. To become a *Weight Loss, God's Way* member, go to:

christianweightlossgodsway.com

Bible Studies for Churches and Small Groups

The membership program can also be experienced a la carte with a group of your friends or with your church. Take one of our three—to-six-week studies on a variety of health and weight-releasing topics. To learn more about starting a Bible study in your home or church, go to:

https://www.cathymorenzie.com/start-a-wlgw-group/

Books and Devotionals

You can find all of our *Healthy by Design* series of weight loss books here:

Christianweightlossbooks.com

Keynote Speaking

Want me to visit your hometown? Need a speaker for your annual conference or special event? My fun and practical approach to *Weight Loss, God's Way* will give your group clarity and focus to move toward their weight loss goals. To learn more or to book a speaking engagement, visit:

https://www.cathymorenzie.com/speaking/

Private Coaching

Prefer a more one-on-one approach? I have a few dedicated time slots available to coach you individually to help you fast-track your results. To learn more, go to:

https://www.cathymorenzie.com/coach-with-cathy-2/

Other Healthy by Design books by Cathy Morenzie:

Weight Loss, God's Way

Healthy Eating, God's Way: 21-Day Meal Plan

Pray Powerfully, Lose Weight

Coming soon:

Breakthrough

Strong Faith, Strong Finish

Online programs by Cathy Morenzie:

Weight Loss, God's Way 21-Day Challenge:
21daysgodsway.com

5 Steps to Christian Weight Loss Course:
5stepscourse.com

Weight Loss, God's Way Membership:
christianweightlossgodsway.com

Love God, Lose Weight:
lovegodloseweight.com

Pray Powerfully, Lose Weight:
praypowerfullyloseweight.com

Strong Faith, Strong Finish:
strongfaithstrongfinish.com

Meet the Authors

Prayers written by Geri Parisella

Geri is a Jesus-loving mom from the Boston area who is a total #wordnerd. You'll find a sudoku book on most of the tables in her house, a Red Sox game on most of the TVs between March and October, and a free-weight or two in her hands most mornings of the week.

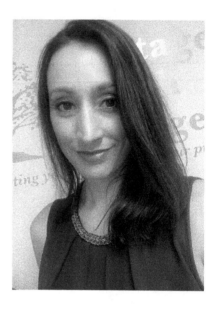

She and her teenaged son—an avid lover of parkour—enjoy spending time together bouncing on their backyard trampoline. They have been blessed to become part of a wonderful church family, where Geri is co-leading an inner-healing ministry.

In the not-too-far-off-future, it wouldn't be surprising to find Geri and her son exploring and adventuring with their family in Europe and elsewhere as they explore the next steps in God's plan for their lives.

Cathy Morenzie

Cathy is a noted personal trainer, author, blogger and presenter, and has been a leader in the faith/fitness industry for over a decade. Her impact has influenced thousands of people over the years to help them lose weight and develop positive attitudes about their bodies and fitness. Over the years, she has seen some of the most powerful and faith-filled people struggle with their health and their weight.

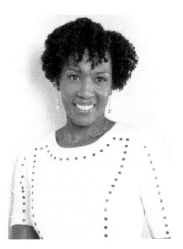

Cathy Morenzie herself—a rational, disciplined, faith-filled personal trainer—struggled with her own weight, emotional eating, self-doubt, and low self-esteem. She tried to change just about everything about herself for much of her life, so she knows what it's like to feel stuck. Every insecurity, challenge, and negative emotion that she experienced has equipped her to help other people who face the same struggles—especially women.

With her Healthy by Design books and Weight Loss, God's Way programs, Cathy has helped thousands to learn to let go of their mental, emotional, and spiritual bonds that have kept them stuck, and instead rely on their Heavenly Father for true release from their fears, doubts, stress, and anxiety. She also teaches people how to eat a sustainable, nutritious diet, and find the motivation to exercise.

Learn more at www.cathymorenzie.com.

Follow Cathy at:
https://www.facebook.com/weightlossgodsway/
https://www.youtube.com/user/activeimage1

Printed in the USA
CPSIA information can be obtained
at www.ICGtesting.com
LVHW051032060324
773716LV00004B/99